# You Must Wash Your Hands

## by
## Karen James

Rev. date: 08/29/2013

To order additional copies of this book, contact:
Xlibris LLC
1-888-795-4274
www.Xlibris.com
Orders@Xlibris.com

The "You Must" books are a series of books promoting
good manners and proper hygiene for little children
everywhere.

Illustrations by Steven Gourgue
Book Design, George Michael Rodrigues

# Dedication

For Almira my inspiration, because of you all of this is possible. You make me happy when skies are grey.

My mother Lesley Patrick I would not be here without you. I thank you and love you from the bottom of my heart.

Mr. Ash Cash, when it was just a dream you told me to make it my reality and though I took my own sweet time I finally did it.

Stevens your illustrations brought this book to life! With my vision and your talent we made this possible. Thank you for your time and energy.

And lastly Jarice James who refused to let me procrastinate any longer. Who believed in any dream I had no matter the size. I love you with all my heart and I am happy that you have motivated me to finish what I started.

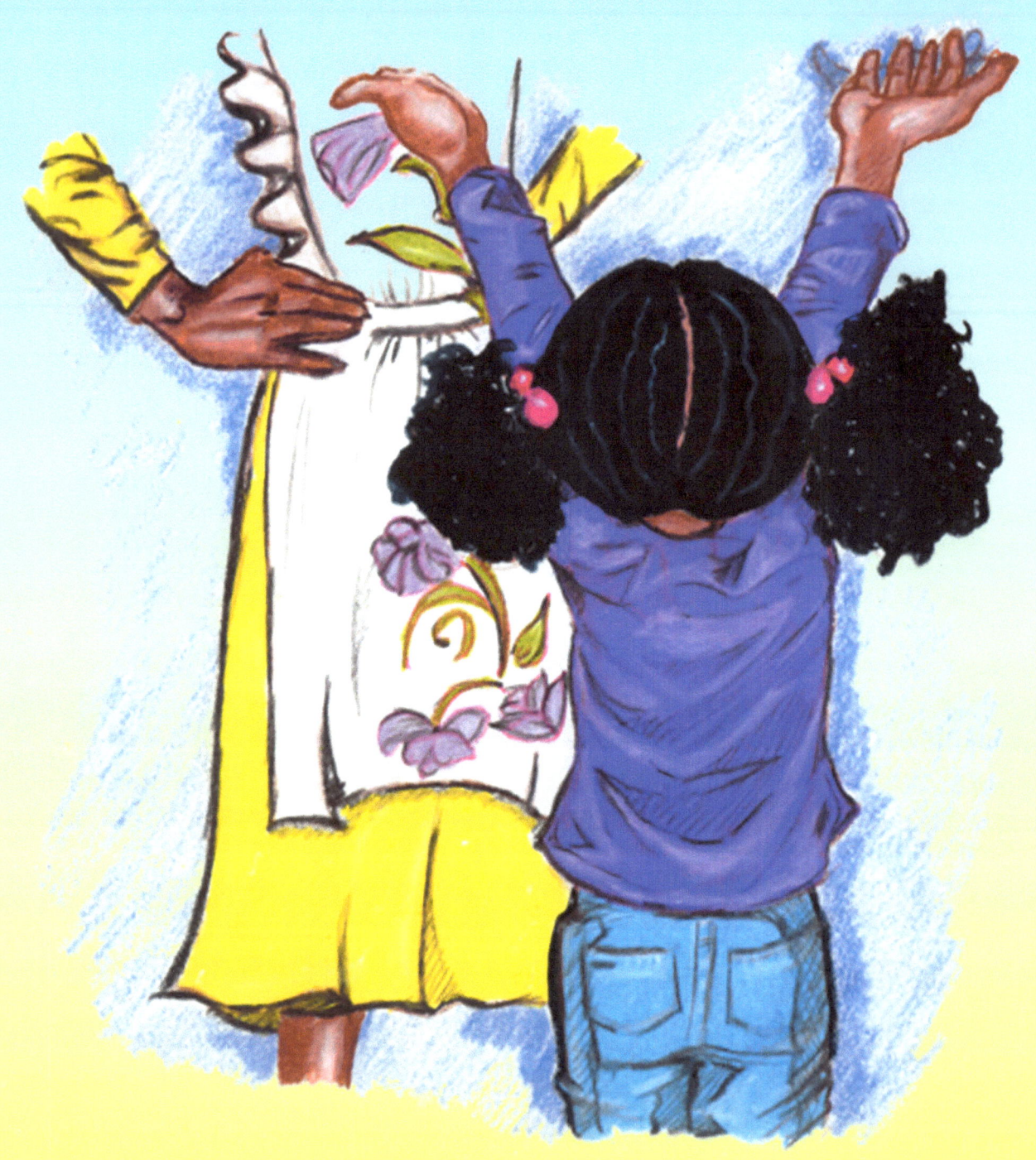

4

Here we go again, you must wash your hands,

Especially since you've been playing in sand.

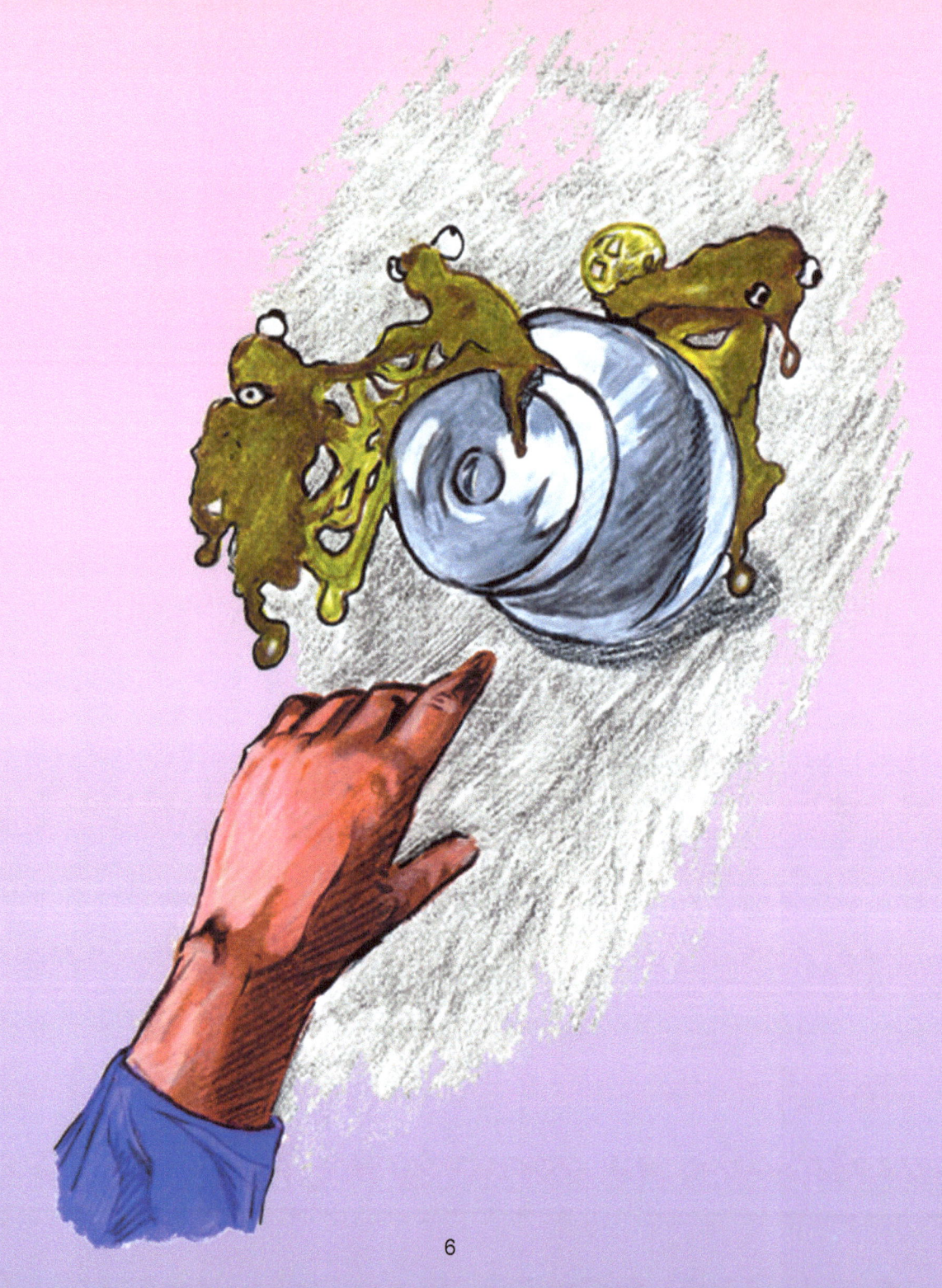

6

You've touched every door knob, the table and chairs,

You've held on to railings while going upstairs.

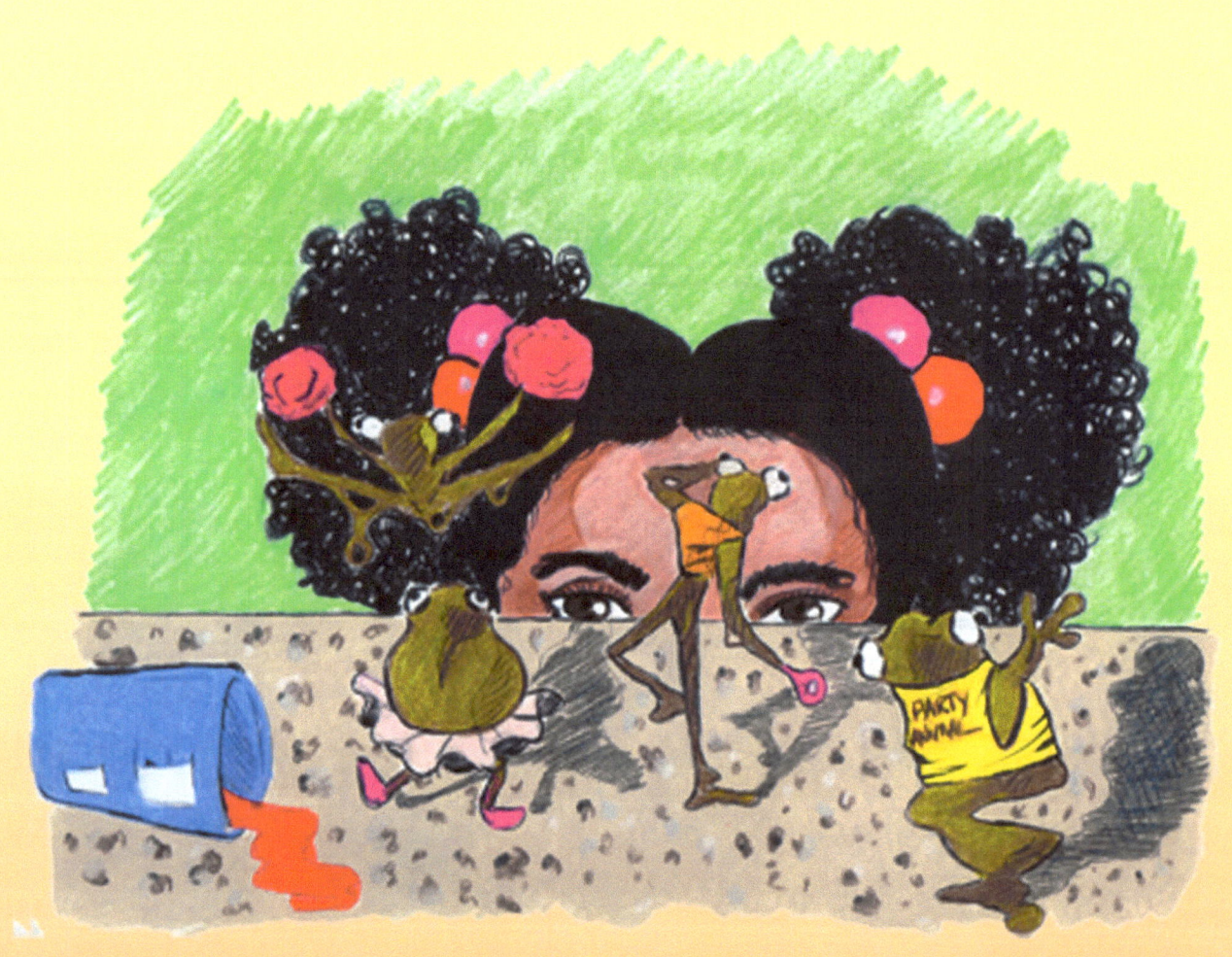

They're all over now all over your hands,

    They're having a ball they're having a dance.

They're getting much bigger in number and size,

    They're spreading and growing in front of our eyes.

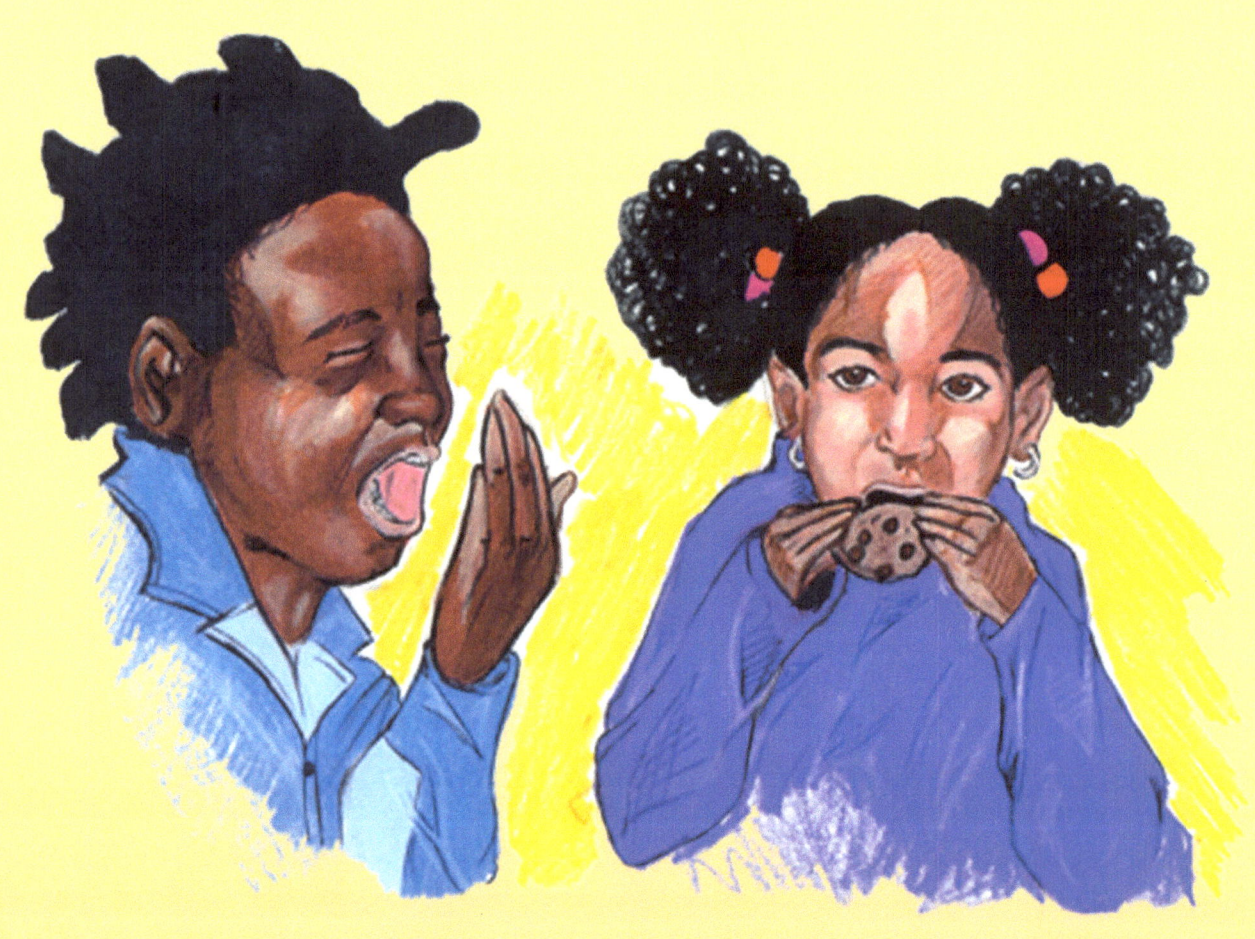

You gave some to Tristan he gave them right back,
You must wash your hands before you have that snack.

"But mommy how can I get rid of them now,
Can you please tell me, can you show me how?"

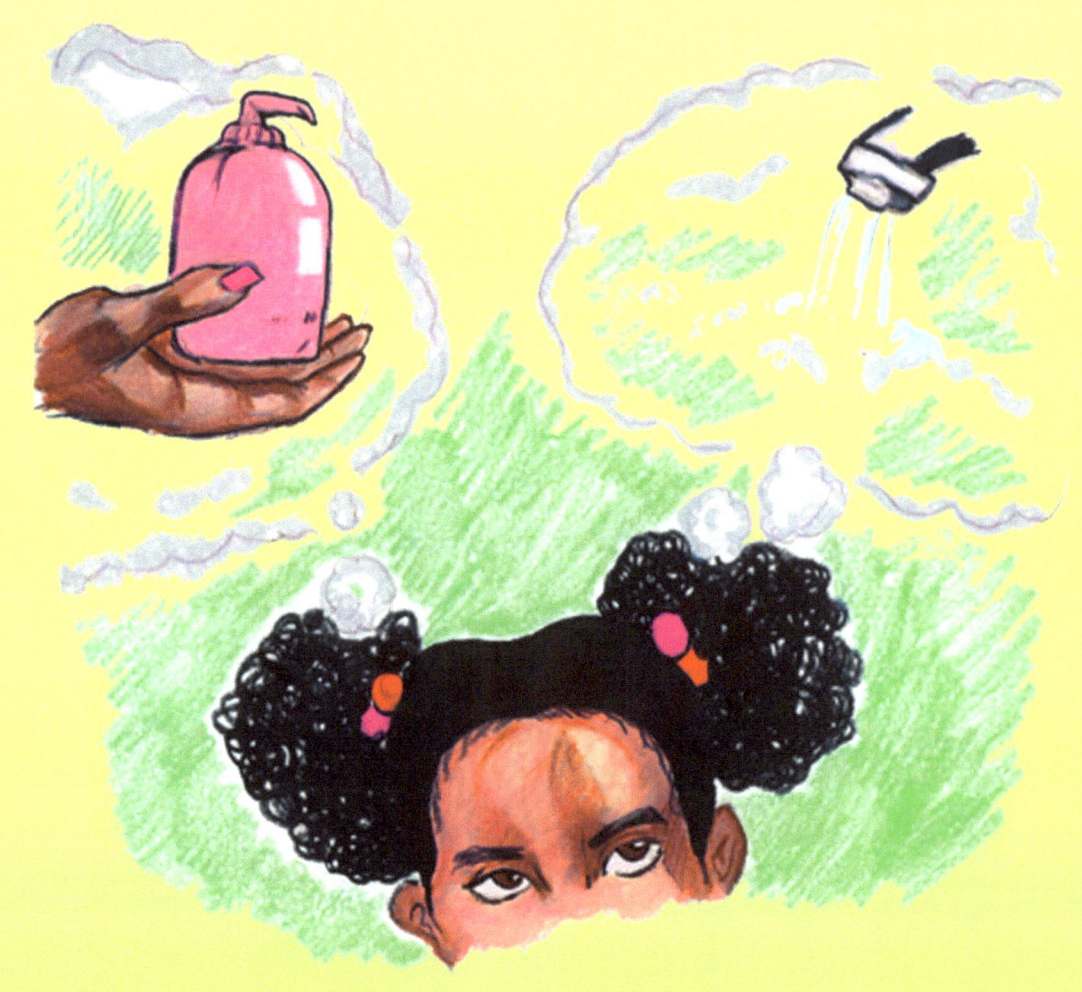

It's very simple just follow these rules,

   And make sure you have your hand washing tools.

Some soap and water will do the trick,

   Because if you don't do this you can get very sick.

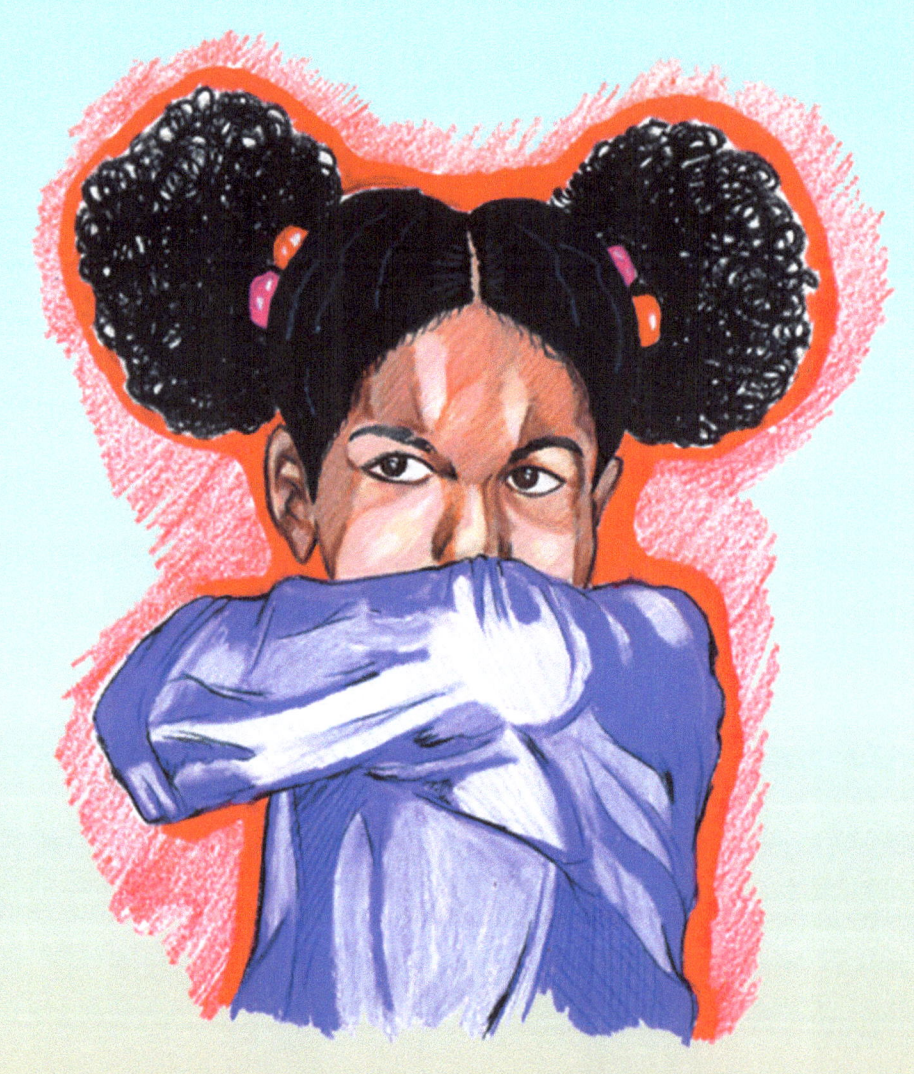

You must wash your hands before every meal,
nice and squeaky clean that's how it should feel

You must was your hands after wiping your nose,
no more rubbing them on your clothes.

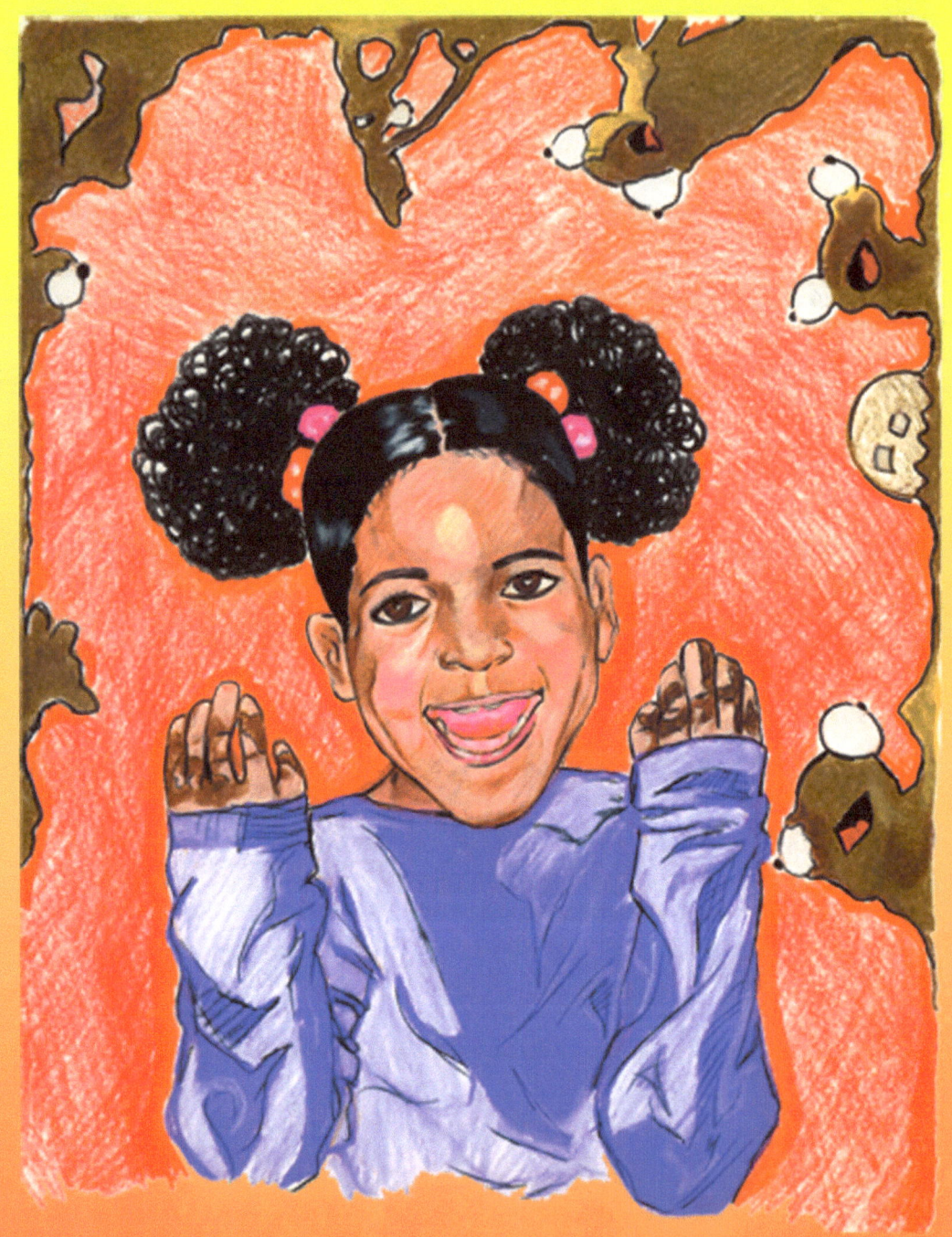

You must wash your hands after each bathroom break, especially now that you know what's at stake

You must tell your friends keep them clean as can be, because we don't like germs but they love you and me

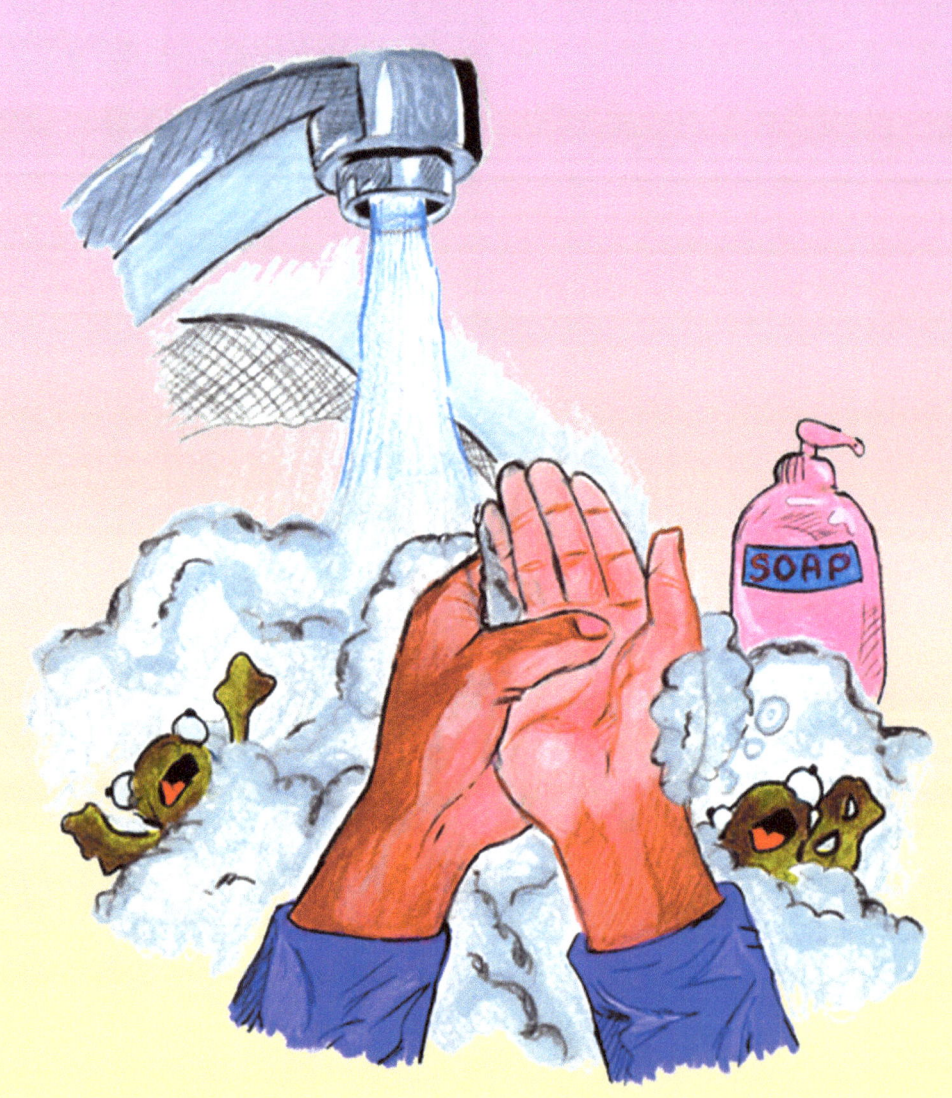

You must wash your hands tell all that you see,

And hope that they'll listen because knowledge is key

You must wash your hands when play time is done,

And wash them away until there are none.

## About the Author

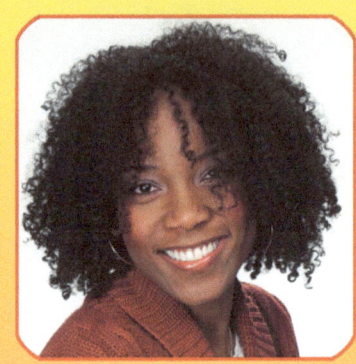

Karen James was born in the beautiful island Dominica and grew up in St. Vincent. Being raised as an only child, her imagination was always running wild. As a teenager she moved to Chicago and realized that her passion for helping and working with children, paired with her vivid imagination made for the perfect combination of writing children stories.

She currently resides in Brooklyn NY where her 4 yr old daughter Amira has inspired her to get the ball rolling on her dream. Having written poetry throughout high school, it came easy for her to write the "You Must" series and being a parent helped quite a bit. In this series of books, she goes to address everyday challenges including proper hygiene and manners that our children encounter, by making it fun and educational at the same time.

She is now in the process of establishing her nonprofit organization I.P.M.D (Interactive Parents Making a Difference). It's an organization designed to encourage other Parents to become more active participants in the upbringing of their children, besides the regular provisions necessary for survival.

And with that, she hopes to make a difference in all of the lives of the children around her and beyond.

Stay tuned for these upcoming books in the "You Must" series by Karen James.

**You Must Brush Your Teeth**

**You Must Clean That Mess**

**You Must Go To Bed**

**You Must Take a Bath**

www.ingramcontent.com/pod-product-compliance
Lightning Source LLC
Chambersburg PA
CBHW060829290526
45792CB00005BB/1853